The Sh
St

Mark Greener spent a ...cuical research before joining *MIMS Magazine* .ui uPs in 1989. Since then, he has written on health and biology for magazines worldwide for patients, healthcare professionals and scientists. He is a member of the Royal Society of Biology and is the author of 21 other books, including *The Heart Attack Survival Guide* (2012) and *The Holistic Health Handbook* (2013), both published by Sheldon Press. Mark lives with his wife, three children and two cats in a Cambridgeshire village.

Sheldon Short Guides

A list of titles in the Overcoming Common Problems series is also available from Sheldon Press, 36 Causton Street, London SW1P 4ST and on our website at www.sheldonpress.co.uk

Asthma
Mark Greener

Depression
Dr Tim Cantopher

Diabetes
Mark Greener and Christine Craggs-Hinton

Heart Attacks
Mark Greener

Liver Disease
Mark Greener

Memory Problems
Dr Sallie Baxendale

Phobias and Panic
Professor Kevin Gournay

Stroke Recovery
Mark Greener

Worry and Anxiety
Dr Frank Tallis

THE SHELDON
SHORT GUIDE TO
STROKE
RECOVERY

Mark Greener

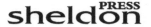

First published in Great Britain in 2016

Sheldon Press
36 Causton Street
London SW1P 4ST
www.sheldonpress.co.uk

British Library Cataloguing-in-Publication Data
A catalogue record for this book is available from the
British Library

ISBN 978–1–84709–401–8
eBook ISBN 978–1–84709–402–5

Typeset by Fakenham Prepress Solutions, Fakenham,
Norfolk NR21 8NN
First printed in Great Britain by Ashford Colour Press
Subsequently digitally reprinted in Great Britain

eBook by Fakenham Prepress Solutions, Fakenham,
Norfolk NR21 8NN

Produced on paper from sustainable forests

Contents

A note to the reader

This is not a medical book and is not intended to replace advice from your doctor. Consult your stroke team, pharmacist or doctor if you believe you have any of the symptoms described, and if you think you might need medical help.

A note on references

I used numerous medical and scientific papers to write the book that this Sheldon Short is based on: *The Stroke Survival Guide*. Unfortunately, there isn't space to include references in this short summary. You can find these in *The Stroke Survival Guide*, which discusses the topics in more detail. I updated some facts and figures for this book.

Introduction

The Stroke Association (<www.stroke.org.uk>) says that there are about 152,000 strokes a year in the UK – one every three-and-a-half minutes. Modern treatments mean that more people survive and recover more fully than before. Nevertheless, a quarter of strokes prove fatal within a year. Indeed, in 2012, strokes were the fourth leading cause of death among men in England and Wales, and the third leading cause among women. Furthermore, half the survivors have some disability often affecting tasks most of us take for granted – such as walking, bathing, dressing, eating and using the toilet.

Your recovery partly depends on your commitment and that of your partner or other carers. You will need to practise exercises, learn to live within any disability, perhaps deal with altered relationships, and make lifestyle changes. People who survive a stroke – even a 'mini-stroke', also called a transient ischaemic attack (TIA) – are much more likely to suffer another, a heart attack or other cardiovascular (heart and blood vessel) diseases. Combining medicines and lifestyle changes can reduce the risk of cardiovascular diseases by four-fifths over five years.

Sometimes a stroke leaves hidden disabilities, such as problems with memory, thinking or concentration, depression and anxiety, and personality changes. The 'sympathy', help and support that survivors and their carers receive is often much less for these hidden problems than for physical disabilities. Not surprisingly, carers are prone to stress, anxiety and depression and may receive little help and advice. So, I hope that this book also supports spouses, family members and other carers. I wish you well.

Get help as soon as possible

Nineteen in every 20 strokes begin outside hospital, and the sooner you act the better the chances of a full recovery. Call 999 or go to the local accident and emergency department if you or someone around you experiences any of the following:

- Weakness or numbness in the face, arm or leg (Can the person smile? Has his or her eye or mouth dropped? Can he or she raise both arms?)
- Loss or slurring of speech (Can the person speak clearly and understand what you say?)
- Loss or blurring of vision
- A sensation of motion (vertigo)
- Difficulty with balance
- Unusual, sudden or severe headache.

1

Your remarkable brain

Strokes occur when the brain's blood supply is blocked. Your brain accounts for about 2 per cent of your weight but uses about 20 per cent of your body's glucose (the sugar that fuels the body). During most strokes, brain cells don't get enough oxygen, glucose and other nutrients and so die. The effects on the body or mind depend on the site of the damage (Figure 1 overleaf):

- Damage to a part of the brain that controls movement can cause 'motor problems', such as weakness, poor dexterity, painful muscle spasms and abnormal postures.
- Damage to the part that processes information can cause 'cognitive impairment': the survivor is less able to think clearly, remember things, solve problems and plan.
- Damage to areas that ensure that you breathe, that your heart beats and that you digest food can prove fatal.

A stroke's effects also depend on the extent of the damage. You may not even realize that you have had a very mild stroke or TIA. Extensive damage can be fatal or occasionally result in:

- vegetative state, where the survivor is awake but does not show any signs of awareness;
- locked-in syndrome, where the survivor is conscious and aware, but paralysed.

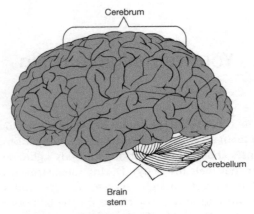

Figure 1 The main areas of the brain

The brainstem, for example, ensures that our basic biological functions – such as breathing, heart rate and swallowing – continue without us thinking about them, even when we are asleep. The brainstem also helps with vision, hearing, balance, movement, the sleep–wake cycle, alertness and keeping our body temperature constant. Strokes that damage a large part of the brainstem can prove fatal or leave the survivor in a vegetative state. Even damage to a small part of the brainstem can cause debilitating problems with, for example, vision, balance and swallowing as well as weak or numb face or limbs.

The cerebellum controls timing and patterns of movement, and aids balance and coordination. It stores patterns of muscle movements – used, for example, when you take part in sport or play an instrument – and helps maintain posture. So, a stroke that damages the cerebellum can cause unsteadiness, poor coordination and clumsiness.

The cerebrum analyses information received from the rest of the body, including our senses, compares our situation with our knowledge and experience, decides if we need to act and sends messages to our muscles. Each of the cerebrum's two hemispheres controls the opposite side. So, a stroke that damages the right hemisphere affects movement on the left side. In most people, the right hemisphere also:

- recognizes shapes, angles, proportions, patterns, faces and so on;
- controls emotions, creativity and imagination;
- is responsible for your awareness of your body.

The left hemisphere oversees analytical thought, problem solving, language, speech and understanding. A thick cord of nerves connects the hemispheres – one reason why the brain sometimes compensates for a stroke's effects: the other hemisphere takes over.

The brain's blood system

The heart's four chambers – two atria and two ventricles (Figure 2 overleaf) – beat in sequence, pushing blood around two circulatory systems that begin and end at the heart (Figure 3 overleaf):

- the pulmonary circulation, which connects your heart to your lungs;
- the systemic circulation, which connects your heart to all other parts of your body.

The atria collect blood from the pulmonary and systemic circulations and push blood into the ventricles. Rapid, uncoordinated beating of the atria (atrial fibrillation) is an important cause of stroke.

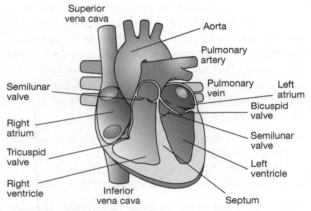

Figure 2 The structure of the heart

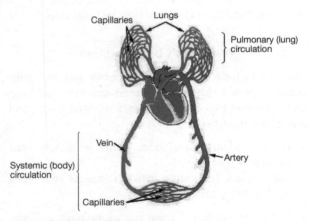

Figure 3 The circulatory system

Go with the flow

Heart valves ensure that blood flows in the correct direction:

- The tricuspid valve controls blood flow between the right atrium and the right ventricle.
- The bicuspid (mitral) valve controls the flow between the left atrium and left ventricle.
- Semilunar valves prevent blood in the arteries from flowing back into the ventricles.

Occasionally, a clot (a 'thrombus') forms on these valves. Fragments of these clots can lodge in the cerebral circulation, potentially triggering a stroke.

2

Causes and types of stroke

Strokes are sudden, seemingly random – 'the stroke of God's hand' according to a sixteenth-century book. And they can strike at any age. Three-quarters occur in people over 65 years of age. But 1 in every 20,000 children in the UK has a stroke each year. While almost everyone's at risk, some people are especially vulnerable:

- People from African Caribbean backgrounds are about twice as likely to have a stroke as white people and tend to have strokes at a younger age. Dangerously raised blood pressure (hypertension), diabetes and sickle cell disease increase stroke risk and are especially common in African Caribbean people.
- People in the most deprived parts of the UK are around three times more likely to die prematurely from a stroke than those in the most affluent areas, partly because of a less healthy diet and higher levels of smoking and stress.
- Men are about 25 per cent more likely to suffer a stroke than women. However, women usually live longer. So, overall, more women suffer a stroke than men.

Types of stroke

There are two main types of stroke:

- About 85 per cent of strokes are ischaemic. An interruption or reduction in the blood supply starves the brain of oxygen and nutrients. Cells supplied by that vessel die.
- About 15 per cent of strokes are intracerebral (inside the head) haemorrhages. A vessel bursts and blood floods into, and destroys, part of the brain.

As we'll see, numerous causes underlie ischaemic and haemorrhagic strokes. But about 12 per cent of strokes are cryptogenic: doctors can't identify the cause. A third of strokes in younger adults are cryptogenic.

Transient ischaemic attacks (TIAs) – heed the mini-stroke warning

Each year, one person in 1,000 has a TIA: a short-lived blood clot interrupts blood flow to part of the brain or the eye:

- When a TIA affects the blood supply to the light-sensitive layer at the back of the eye (retina), the person can experience temporary blindness in one eye.
- When the TIA affects the blood supply to the brain, he or she can develop typical signs of a stroke.

About half of people referred to a specialist with a suspected TIA turn out to have another condition, such as migraine, a brain tumour or multiple sclerosis.

The body restores the blood supply relatively rapidly. So, TIA symptoms often last only a few minutes, resolve within 24 hours and do not produce long-lasting problems. Nevertheless, many persistent changes produced by a mild stroke are subtle and doctors treat TIAs in essentially the same way. So, the exact border between a TIA and mild stroke isn't always clear.

Occasionally, an embolism or a small haemorrhage causes a TIA. Usually, however, a TIA or mild stroke is a warning that you have atherosclerosis in the blood vessels to your brain. Over time, atherosclerosis can worsen and, eventually, you could suffer a devastating stroke. Indeed, about one person in 50 who experiences a TIA has a stroke within the next two days, with 1 in 20 having a stroke within seven days. The stroke risk is especially high if you:

- experience crescendo TIA – more than two episodes in a week;
- have atrial fibrillation (page 16);
- are taking anticoagulants (blood thinning drugs).

Treating TIA urgently prevents four in five of these strokes. So, don't dismiss symptoms as fatigue, a trapped nerve, migraine or a funny turn. Call 999 or ask someone to drive you to A&E as soon as you develop any symptoms that might indicate a stroke (page xii).

Ischaemic strokes

A build-up of fat (athersclerosis) inside the arteries supplying the brain causes about half of ischaemic strokes. As a plaque enlarges, the lumen (the 'bore' down the middle of the vessel) narrows (Figure 4). The bigger the vessel, the greater the area of brain supplied and, as a rule, the greater the risk of death and disability. Atherosclerosis can form in the vessels supplying a relatively small area. But if this includes a critical area, a small stroke can still be devastating.

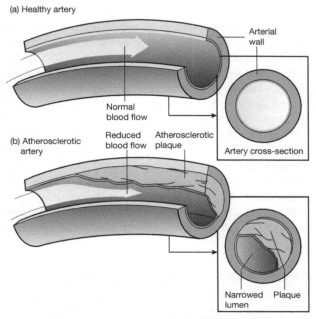

Figure 4 Atherosclerotic plaques can narrow the lumen of an artery

Atherosclerosis begins as smears of fat around damage to the blood vessel's normally smooth inner lining caused by, for example:

- excessive levels of fat in the blood (dyslipidaemia);
- raised sugar levels in the blood (diabetes);
- hypertension;
- age-related changes to blood vessels;
- nicotine and other toxins from smoking.

The damage allows fats and white blood cells (which normally fight infections) to enter the vessel wall and trigger changes that 'patch' the damage. But it's a short-term 'fix'. Fat continues to pour into the plaque. Over time, muscle cells cover a core of fat-engorged blood cells, fat and debris from dead cells. Capillaries grow into the developing plaque: but they're fragile and blood leaks into, and further swells, the plaque. Calcium accumulates in, and gradually hardens, the plaque.

At first, arteries enlarge to compensate. But after the plaque occupies more than 40 per cent of the vessel wall, the lumen narrows and blood flow falls. The plaques can burst, triggering a blood clot that may block the vessel and cause an ischaemic stroke or TIA (Figure 5). The process is the same as that causing most heart attacks. In TIAs, the body dissolves the clot before enough brain cells die to cause irreversible problems.

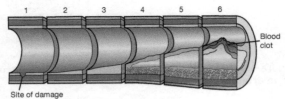

Site of damage
1 Damage to the inner lining of the blood vessel
2 Fatty streak forms at site of damage
3 Numbers of white blood cells increase, area is inflamed and small pools of fat appear
4 Large core of fat develops, and amounts of muscle and collagen increase
5 Fibrous cap covers a fat-rich core, while calcium deposits harden the plaque
6 Plaque ruptures, triggering a blood clot

Figure 5 Development of an atherosclerotic plaque

An ischaemic stroke produces two 'zones' of damage:

- In the 'core' zone, a dramatic decline in blood flow rapidly kills brain cells.
- The penumbra refers to the area between regions with a normal blood supply and the core zone. Cells

in the penumbra receive blood from surrounding vessels. While these cells survive for a few minutes to several hours, they eventually die if the blood supply does not return to normal.

Rapid treatment restores the blood supply, which reduces the size of the penumbra – and, therefore, the risk of brain damage.

Embolism

In up to a third of ischaemic strokes, a fragment of a blood clot (thromboembolism) blocks an artery supplying the brain. For example:

- Atrial fibrillation (page 16) can leave blood in the heart, which can clot. Fragments can break off, forming an embolism that can travel to and block arteries supplying the brain.
- Embolisms can arise from a deep vein thrombosis (DVT), which occurs when a blood clot forms in a vein in the lower leg, thigh, pelvis or, less commonly, the arm. Fragments of the clot can cause ischaemic strokes or travel to the lungs, causing a blockage called a pulmonary embolism – an important cause of death after a stroke.

Haemorrhagic strokes

Haemorrhagic strokes are, generally, more severe and cause more deaths than ischaemic strokes. During a haemorrhagic stroke, a blood vessel supplying the brain bursts. Blood floods into the brain. A very small amount of blood (micro-bleed) usually does not cause symptoms – doctors identify them only on a brain scan for another reason. However, people who have micro-bleeds are more likely to have a full-blown haemorrhagic stroke. A large haemorrhagic stroke can rapidly kill.

Haemorrhagic strokes have three main causes:

- weakened or damaged blood vessels – such as an aneurysm;
- blood that does not clot properly;
- hypertension.

Subarachnoid haemorrhage

The membranes (meninges) covering the brain and spinal cord consist of three layers:

- the pia mater, closest to the brain or spinal cord;
- the dura mater, just under the skull or next to the bones in the spine; and
- the arachnoid layer, between the pia mater and the dura mater.

During a subarachnoid haemorrhage, blood accumulates in the space beneath the arachnoid layer. About a quarter of people with subarachnoid haemorrhage die within 24 hours. Half the survivors are disabled. Again, rapid treatment improves your prospects. So, call 999 if you experience any of the following:

- sudden agonizing headache – like being suddenly hit on the head;
- stiff neck;
- nausea and vomiting that you cannot explain;
- over-sensitivity to light;
- blurred or double vision;
- confusion;
- other stroke symptoms, such as slurred speech and weakness on one side of the body;

- unconsciousness;
- convulsions (uncontrollable shaking).

Aneurysm

Most subarachnoid haemorrhages occur when a cerebral aneurysm bursts. Usually cerebral aneurysms – a 'pouch' or 'ballooning' of an artery, often where the vessel's lining is weak – do not cause symptoms. However, some aneurysms burst, such as when blood pressure reaches a short-lived peak, during, for example, strong emotions, heavy lifting, coughing, sex and even urination and defecation. The initial bleed may last only seconds. But further bleeding is common and, if persistent, can lead to coma and death.

Aneurysms can form elsewhere. For example, weak heart muscle can form a 'pocket' called a ventricular aneurysm. Clots and, in turn, embolisms can form in these pockets.

Surgery can strengthen aneurysms. For instance, if you have two or more close relatives (parent, sibling or child) who have an aneurysm or if you have polycystic renal disease you are at increased risk of having an aneurysm. Talk to your GP to see if it is worth being screened and, if you have an aneurysm, discuss the risks and benefits of surgery.

3

Risk factors for stroke

Hypertension

Hypertension, which contributes to about half of strokes, rarely causes symptoms. But see a doctor urgently if you suffer any symptom in Table 1, which could be a sign of an especially dangerous form of raised blood pressure called malignant hypertension.

Over time, hypertension changes blood vessels' structure. For example, the vessels' walls become thicker, stronger and stiffer. These changes reduce the risk of damage but tend to maintain high blood pressure and, eventually, the vessels become more brittle. So, a sudden increase in blood pressure from exercise or emotion can burst a blood vessel, causing a haemorrhagic stroke. Hypertension can damage the arteries' smooth inner lining, sowing the seed for

Table 1 Symptoms that could indicate malignant hypertension

Confusion

Changes in vision

Fatigue

Headache – especially if severe

Irregular heartbeat

Nosebleed, without injury

Tinnitus (unexplained buzzing or noise in the ears)

atherosclerosis, or trigger a plaque to burst, resulting in an ischaemic stroke. Even increases in blood pressure that are only just above normal – so-called pre-hypertension – might contribute to up to a fifth of strokes. So, if you have had a stroke or are at increased risk, discuss treating pre-hypertension with your doctor.

Doctors can identify a cause for, at most, one in ten cases of hypertension. These causes include:

- some kidney diseases;
- drinking too much alcohol;
- eating too much salt, or being abnormally sensitive to salt;
- being overweight.

Treating the cause often lowers blood pressure to safe levels. In other people, drugs (antihypertensives) and lifestyle changes can reduce blood pressure. However, antihypertensives are added to – and not a replacement for – lifestyle changes.

A doctor or nurse should measure your blood pressure at least once a year. You can buy blood pressure monitors to use at home. However, make sure the monitor is accurate and you have the right-sized cuff. Your GP or hospital, the British Heart Foundation (<www.bhf.org.uk>) or Blood Pressure UK (<www.bloodpressureuk.org>) may be able to help.

Lethal and healthy cholesterol

Cholesterol, a type of fat, is a building block of the membranes that surround every cell, forms part of the myelin sheath around many nerves that ensures that signals travel properly and is the backbone of several hormones. Unfortunately, many of us have too much of a good thing.

Blood is about four-fifths water. Fat and water do not mix. So, your body surrounds the core of cholesterol with a coat of special chemicals called 'lipoproteins'. For example:

- Low-density lipoprotein (LDL) carries cholesterol from the liver to the tissues. LDL accumulates in artery walls, which contributes to atherosclerosis.
- High-density lipoprotein (HDL) carries cholesterol from the arteries to the liver for removal. So, HDL removes cholesterol from plaques, slowing atherosclerosis.

In other words, high LDL levels increase stroke risk. High HDL levels protect. It's easy to remember: LDL is 'lethal'; HDL is 'healthy'. Fat is a concentrated source of energy – one gram provides nine calories. So, a high-fat diet can contribute to people being overweight or obese, another risk factor for stroke.

Arrhythmias

Usually the heart beats regularly and steadily, the pace changing to keep up with the demands we face. Sometimes, however, the heartbeat becomes irregular – a so-called arrhythmia. Most arrhythmias are harmless, but some are serious or even life-threatening.

For example, in atrial fibrillation, the atria beat irregularly and rapidly, quiver (fibrillate) and only partly contract. Furthermore, the contractions of the atria and ventricles are uncoordinated. Because the heart pumps less effectively, people with atrial fibrillation may experience breathlessness, palpitations and dizziness. The poorly coordinated contractions can leave blood in the heart, where it can clot and embolize. Indeed, atrial fibrillation might cause up to a quarter of strokes.

Everyone who has an irregular pulse should have an ECG whether or not they experience symptoms. You should also have your pulse taken if you experience breathlessness, palpitations or dizziness. If you have atrial fibrillation, explore the treatments with your doctor.

Clots on heart valves

Clots can form if the heart valves are:

- misshapen – for example, because of developmental problems in the womb;
- scarred – for example, from rheumatic heart disease; or artificial (after valve-replacement surgery).

For instance, in 'mitral valve prolapse', the bicuspid valve dips deeply into the ventricle. Mitral valve prolapse does not usually cause problems. Occasionally, however, the valve can be the site of a clot.

Arterial dissection

Violent movements or neck injuries – such as from a car accident – can damage the carotid or vertebral arteries. So, blood can get inside the layers that make up the blood vessel wall. This pushes the sides of the vessel together and blocks the flow. In other cases, damage to the smooth inner lining of the vessel increases the chance that a clot will form. This damage, which doctors call arterial dissection, tends to occur in young people.

Heart attacks

If you have atherosclerosis in one part of your body, you probably have plaques elsewhere, such as in the blood vessels supplying your heart. Each year, about one person in 50 who has survived a TIA or stroke experiences a heart attack. And up to one person in 20 who has a heart attack has a stroke. For example, emboli can arise from clots on the dead muscle in the heart. Some people – especially the elderly and those with diabetes – can experience relatively painless heart attacks. A stroke might be the first sign that they have suffered a heart attack.

Sickle cell anaemia

Sickle cell anaemia – a genetic disease that causes crescent-shaped red blood cells (erythrocytes) – is most common in people of African heritage and seems to protect against malaria. The crescent-shaped erythrocytes can, however, clump inside blood vessels, increasing stroke risk. Indeed, children with sickle cell disease are between 200 and 400 times more likely to have a stroke than those without the condition. Blood transfusions replace sickle cells with normally shaped erythrocytes and, therefore, cut stroke risk.

Polycythaemia

People with polycythaemia produce too many erythrocytes. This thickens the blood, which cannot circulate easily. In addition, erythrocytes can clump, causing strokes, pulmonary embolisms and heart attacks. Regularly removing about a pint of blood and taking drugs to slow erythrocyte production help treat polycythaemia.

Diabetes

Cells use glucose as fuel. The body extracts glucose from carbohydrates (such as starch and sugars) that we eat. Insulin stimulates cells to take glucose from the blood. Some people with diabetes don't produce enough insulin. In others, insulin does not work properly when it reaches cells (insulin resistance). (Some people show both changes.) So, cells do not absorb enough glucose and blood sugar levels rise.

Dangerously high blood sugar levels (hyperglycaemia) slowly poison cells, potentially causing, for example, pain, ulcers, amputations, heart disease and blindness. In addition, people with diabetes are twice as likely as other people to have a stroke in the five years after their doctor has diagnosed diabetes. Atherosclerosis accounts for most of this increased risk.

Legal and illegal drugs

Smoking and alcohol are among the most important risk factors for stroke:

- Smoking directly causes almost one in five strokes.
- A person smoking 20 cigarettes a day is six times more likely to suffer a stroke than a non-smoker.
- A smoker with hypertension is 20 times more likely to have a stroke than a non-smoker with normal blood pressure.
- Heavy drinkers are about three times more likely to suffer a stroke than those who drink sensibly.

● Illicit drugs can also cause strokes. For instance, users were six to seven times more likely to suffer an ischaemic stroke within 24 hours of taking cocaine. Moreover, cocaine, amphetamines, ecstasy and some other drugs can markedly increase blood pressure. So, blood vessels may rupture, especially if the person has an aneurysm or another cardiovascular weakness.

If you know someone who abuses legal or illegal drugs ask him or her, gently, non-confrontationally and without condemning his or her use, to seek help from the GP (see also pages 51 and 54). In the case of illegal drugs, users can contact their local drug services (see NHS Choices, <www.nhs.uk>) or the advice service Frank (<www.talktofrank.com>). Do not assume 'legal highs' are risk-free. Scientific studies have examined relatively few legal highs.

Stress and depression

Stress seems to increase stroke risk. Bereavement is, for example, extremely stressful. Stroke risk more than doubles in the first 30 days after people lose their partner. Anger is a common reaction to stress. The risk of an ischaemic stroke may be up to eight-fold higher, and an aneurysm is about six times more likely to burst, in the two hours after an angry outburst.

Stress contributes to depression, which increases stroke risk by about a third. Depressed people are, for example, less likely to eat healthily and are more likely to 'self-medicate' with tobacco, alcohol and illicit drugs, all of which increase stroke risk. In turn, stroke seems to increase the risk of depression, both as a reaction to the life-changing event and following damage to brain areas that regulate emotion.

Infections

Several infections, including syphilis, HIV, shingles and influenza, increase stroke risk. For example, strokes are more common during the winter, partly because influenza is widespread. The flu jab cuts stroke risk by about a quarter. The reduction is strongest with vaccinations early in the flu season. So, get the jab as soon as you can each year.

The varicella-zoster virus (VZV) causes chickenpox. After you recover from chickenpox, VZV can 'hide' in nerves. Physical and emotional stress, some medicines, age and so on can reactivate VZV, which moves along the nerves into the skin, where it causes shingles. Occasionally, VZV moves along the nerves to the head where its re-emergence can trigger TIAs and strokes. Antiviral medicines 'attack' VZV and reduce stroke risk.

Pregnancy and the pill

Women who develop pre-eclampsia (hypertension and high levels of protein in their urine during pregnancy) are twice as likely to have a stroke and four times more likely to develop hypertension in later life than mothers-to-be whose blood pressure remains normal.

The pill causes one extra ischaemic stroke per year for every 20,000 women using low-dose oestrogen oral contraceptives. In general, oral contraceptives or hormone replacement therapy increase stroke risk only in women with other risk factors, such as migraines or hypertension. If you have other risk factors or a history of TIA or stroke, discuss other hormonal and non-hormonal contraceptives with your doctor or nurse.

4

Diagnosing and treating stroke

Modern treatments used quickly dramatically increase your chances of surviving a stroke and avoiding serious disability – but doctors need to get the diagnosis right. Unfortunately, several illnesses can mimic strokes, and haemorrhagic and ischaemic strokes can cause the same symptoms. Even today, about a fifth of stroke diagnoses made in a typical accident and emergency department are wrong.

Brain scans

Computed tomography (CT) – previously called computerized axial tomography (CAT) – scans allow doctors to look inside the brain. Almost all stroke patients have a brain scan, although not always within the recommended 24 hours. However, about one person in 100 develops massive bleeding after an ischaemic stroke. This can resemble a haemorrhagic stroke on brain scans. So, the earlier the hospital performs the scan, the better: some live-saving drugs in ischaemic strokes can cause brain haemorrhages.

Doctors may use ultrasound or Doppler scans to investigate the carotid artery. A Doppler scan measures blood cells' speed, which changes if the artery narrows. Your doctor might suggest cerebral angiography.

During cerebral angiography a surgeon moves a thin tube (catheter) to the neck arteries and then injects a dye that shows up on X-ray.

A doctor or nurse will also take a blood sample, which will be used to check, for example:

- the number of red blood cells (see polycythaemia, page 18);
- how long your blood takes to clot;
- your blood glucose level – very low levels can cause symptoms that mimic some strokes.

Clot-busting drugs

People with ischaemic strokes often receive a 'thrombolytic', which breaks down emboli and the clots formed when an atherosclerotic plaque ruptures. Rapid thrombolytic treatment restores blood flow, which limits further damage:

- Each minute saved between the start of symptoms and treatment may preserve two million brain cells.
- Each hour a stroke remains untreated 'ages' the brain by 3.6 years.
- Thrombolysis starting within 90 minutes of the onset of symptoms more than doubles the likelihood that the survivor will recover without disability.

So, call 999 if you or someone around you shows stroke signs (page xii).

Thrombolysis makes it harder for your blood to clot. So, the risk of fatal and non-fatal intracerebral haemorrhages rises within seven days of treatment. In most cases, the benefits outweigh the risks.

Sometimes surgeons use a mechanical 'clot retrieval system' to remove the blockage. They pass a catheter into the top of the leg and into the cerebral blood vessels. The risk of bleeding seems to be similar to thrombolysis.

Anticoagulation

DVTs occur in up to half of stroke survivors. DVTs can cause pulmonary embolisms, which generally occur two to four weeks after the stroke. Anticoagulants (such as heparin or warfarin) can reduce this risk. Heparin works rapidly. So it's usually given first. You might take warfarin (or a newer anticoagulant) to prevent another clot forming,

Warfarin

Doctors treat atrial fibrillation by slowing the heart or reducing the risk of clots. Warfarin can prevent three in every five strokes in people with atrial fibrillation, for example. Warfarin and related drugs (coumarins) interfere with vitamin K, which is needed to clot blood.

Uncontrolled bleeding is warfarin's main side effect. In any year, one person in 20 taking warfarin will have a minor bleed, while one person in 100 will have a serious haemorrhage. Warfarin can interact with many other drugs and some foods. So, tell your doctor and pharmacist about any other drugs you are taking or before making major changes to your diet. You'll need regular tests to see how long your blood takes to clot to help doctors tailor the dose.

Several newer anticoagulants (such as apixaban, dabigatran or rivaroxaban) act more quickly than warfarin, have fewer interactions and do not require intensive monitoring. However, doctors cannot reverse excessive anticoagulation by adding vitamin K, as they can with warfarin, and each drug has a different pattern of side effects. Discuss which is right for you with your doctor.

Aspirin

When you start bleeding, platelets gather at the wound and stick together forming a clot. Aspirin prevents this 'platelet aggregation'. So, aspirin helps prevent emboli and the clots that form when an atherosclerotic plaque ruptures. For example:

- About one extra person remains independent after a stroke for every 100 who take aspirin in the first two weeks after a stroke.
- In people at high risk (for example, following a heart attack or stroke), aspirin reduces the likelihood of stroke, heart attack or death from vascular disease by almost a quarter.
- In people who have already had a stroke, aspirin prevents about one in seven recurrent strokes.

Before you start taking aspirin your doctor will make sure (e.g. using a brain scan) that you haven't had an intracerebral haemorrhage. Never take aspirin – to relieve a headache, for example – if you're using other anticoagulants unless your doctor suggests the combination. You could risk excessive bleeding and even a haemorrhagic stroke.

Several other drugs (such as dipyridamole and clopidogrel) target platelets, which your doctor may suggest, for example if you develop aspirin's side effects. These include upset stomach, indigestion, bruising and bleeding in the stomach. Dipyridamole can cause, among other reactions, diarrhoea, dizziness, nausea, dyspepsia, headache and muscle aches. Clopidogrel can cause diarrhoea and a skin rash and bleeding. So, discuss which is right for you.

Hypertension

Hypertension is a leading cause of strokes and TIAs. A few people can reach safe blood pressures by changing their diet and lifestyle. Nevertheless, most people also need to take at least two blood pressure lowering drugs (antihypertensives). Doctors can choose from numerous antihypertensives. There's not space here to discuss the pros and cons of each. So, talk to your doctor and check out NHS Choices and patient groups' websites.

Cholesterol-lowering drugs

Cholesterol-lowering drugs seem to prevent between one in seven and one in four strokes in people at high risk, while reducing the risk of major coronary events (e.g. a heart attack) by between a quarter and a third. However, statins, the most widely used cholesterol-lowering drugs, can cause several side effects, including: headache; dizziness; changes in the enzymes produced by your liver; rash; and muscle pain and cramps. If you feel unwell while taking statins (or any other drug), see your GP.

Surgery for strokes

Surgery to stop bleeding, relieve the pressure and bypass the burst blood vessel is often the only treatment for haemorrhagic stroke. So, patients with suspected haemorrhagic stroke should see a neurosurgeon as soon as possible, who may also suggest one of several other procedures:

- Carotid endarterectomy, which widens arteries narrowed by an atherosclerotic plaque, usually takes one to two hours under a general or local anaesthetic. The surgeon makes a small cut into your neck and removes the inner lining of the narrowed part of the artery along with any plaque. The benefits are greater the sooner you have carotid endarterectomy after a minor stroke or TIA.
- During angioplasty, the surgeon threads a catheter tipped with a balloon and guided by X-ray to the blockage. Once it is in place, the surgeon inflates the balloon, which compresses the plaque, widens the artery and improves blood flow.
- In some cases, the surgeon slips a 'collapsed' wire-mesh tube called a stent over the catheter. When the surgeon inflates the balloon, the stent expands and remains in place after the balloon deflates. Within a few weeks, the artery's inner lining covers the stent, allowing blood to flow easily without clotting.
- Surgery can repair ruptured areas or reinforce damaged areas to prevent strokes. However, when an aneurysm bursts, muscles in the blood vessels can go into spasm. This spasm, which usually occurs between three and five days after the stroke, narrows the vessel and can further reduce the blood flow to the brain. So, surgeons need to decide whether to operate before the spasms have time to develop or to wait a few weeks for the spasms to subside. You tend to do better if you undergo an operation before the spasms develop. However, 'early' operations are more likely to cause complications. Discuss the risks and benefits with your surgeon.

- Some large ischaemic strokes cause swelling over up to a third of the brain. Untreated, this condition, called 'malignant middle cerebral artery syndrome', kills four in every five people. So, surgeons may remove part of the skull to relieve the pressure. Decompression surgery halves the number of deaths and increases the number of people who survive this syndrome with mild or moderate, rather than severe, disability.

5

Stroke rehabilitation

Stroke rehabilitation aims to ensure that each survivor reaches his or her maximum potential despite any disability (Table 2). So, a multidisciplinary team individualizes your rehabilitation according to your needs and limitations. Most of the improvement in movement, senses and speech occurs three to six months after the stroke. Nevertheless, many survivors

Table 2 Examples of problems after a stroke

Difficulty	Per cent of survivors affected
General movement	80
Altered sensation	Up to 80
Arm movement	70
Problems with sight	Up to 66
Long-term inability to use one arm	40
Altered swallowing (dysphagia)	40
Altered speech (aphasia/dysphasia)	33
Spasticity	19–38
Depression	29
Dementia six months after the stroke	20
Pain after the stroke	5–20
Incontinence a year after the stroke	15

Source: Adapted from the Stroke Association

find that they continue to recover months and years after their stroke, long after formal rehabilitation ends.

The team sets and regularly re-evaluates realistic short- and long-term goals that help you participate in, for example, leisure and family activities. Rehabilitation may target a specific problem, such as weak ankles that make standing and getting around difficult. In other cases, such as washing and dressing, the team may break the activity down. So, the exercise may seem a little divorced from your everyday life. Understanding how it will be of use helps you stay motivated.

You will often have a lot of information to take on board and strokes can undermine memory and cognition. Jotting notes during the consultation and listing your questions can help. Talking over the discussions with your relatives or carers helps consolidate the memory and reveals if there is anything you are unsure about. A quick phone call to the stroke team or to a patient group often resolves any uncertainty.

Get what you are entitled to

Families and stroke survivors may overestimate how well they can cope, especially as support from community health and social services may be limited. You should receive clear advice about your rights, benefits and support. If you do not, ask. A social worker can help you and your carer access the benefits, transport and services that help rehabilitation.

Cognitive impairment

Up to three in five stroke survivors show some impairment in cognition: the ability to think, remember and plan. Indeed, stroke is now the second most common cause of dementia, after Alzheimer's disease. A clinical psychologist can find tailored ways to overcome your particular cognitive problems. You can give your memory a hand by:

- using memory aids – such as lists or a diary;
- fixing a routine – such as mealtimes, or times when relatives or friends call;
- breaking up tasks – such as dressing and cooking – into steps using lists or pictures;
- sticking notes or pictures on important cupboards and drawers – such as where you keep foods, drinks and cutlery;
- craftwork and board games. Craftwork can also help manual dexterity.

Some strokes damage the part of the brain that translates ideas into actions (apraxia). For example, a person with apraxia may not be able to make a cup of tea or use a spoon at the right time. Some people with apraxia can perform the movement when they do not think about it, but not when asked. Apraxia isn't stubbornness or manipulative behaviour.

Language problems

Imagine having a word on the tip of your tongue all the time. That's the problem experienced by many stroke survivors with dysphasia – also called aphasia. For example, survivors may know what they want to say but they can't find the right words (expressive dysphasia). Some cannot call for help or have problems naming objects or people.

Other survivors experience problems understanding what other people say (receptive dysphasia). Others use words incorrectly, speak gibberish or make up words. This 'fluent dysphasia' is often associated with severe problems in understanding.

Around a third of survivors develop dysphasia soon after their stroke. About one in eight show dysphasia six months later. Not surprisingly, speech problems are among the most difficult disabilities to cope with and increase the risk of depression, for carers as well as survivors.

Communication problems can also arise when a stroke damages certain muscles in the face. So, the survivor may have problems forming words (dysarthria). Dysphonia arises when the stroke affects the voice box, causing problems forming words or controlling the volume of the voice.

Even if you have problems talking, try to communicate with other people and not push them away. Communicating helps prevent isolation and loneliness. If you find communication difficult, you or your carer should ask your GP or stroke team for a referral to a speech and language therapist, who will assess and manage the particular problem. For example, the therapist may be able to teach the survivor to use gestures, word-and-picture cards, symbols and computers and smartphone apps to aid communication. Involving survivors in decisions and conversations, even if there are problems understanding or communicating, underscores that they are still part of the family. A growing range of adaptations aid communication: think of Stephen Hawking's eloquence.

Communication aid

If you are speaking to a stroke survivor:

- Do not raise your voice unless you know someone's hearing is poor. If you find you have to raise your voice a lot, check whether he or she needs a hearing aid or if the current device is working properly.
- If you (or the stroke survivor) wear dentures, make sure they still fit properly. This makes speaking easier.
- Do not speak to the survivor as if you are talking to a child. Just because a person cannot speak, that does not mean that he or she does not understand. However, it is worth gently checking that the stroke survivor understands what you are saying, and vice versa.
- Speak slowly. You may sometimes need to repeat what you say. However, try to rephrase things, rather than just saying the same thing over and over.
- Try to establish eye contact. The survivor can watch your face and lips, which helps his or her understanding.
- Listen to the survivor but do not pretend to understand what he or she is saying. This just creates confusion. You could ask the survivor to point or use gestures.
- Resist the temptation to speak for the survivor when you are with family, friends or on a day out.
- Reduce distractions, such as the television or radio, when you are trying to communicate.

Sensory changes

Up to four in every five stroke survivors report sensory changes – such as unpleasant feelings of hot, cold or tingling (pins and needles), and pain – especially if they have motor problems. Therapists typically use two approaches to 're-train' senses.

- Passive re-training uses electrical stimulation to improve function and reduce pain.
- Active re-training repeatedly exposures the survivor to different stimuli, including texture, temperature, joint position or shape.

Difficulty swallowing

Dysphagia (difficulty swallowing), limited arm movement, poor dental hygiene, depression, anxiety, fatigue and unfamiliar foods can contribute to poor nutrition and dehydration, which are common after a stroke. So, when you reach hospital with a suspected stroke, a doctor or nurse will assess your ability to swallow. If you cannot take enough food and water by mouth within 24 hours of reaching hospital, you may need a nasogastric tube, which runs from your nose into your stomach. An experienced professional – such as speech and language therapist or dietician – will assess your swallowing ability in detail once you are out of immediate danger. In addition, watch for:

- difficulty controlling food in the mouth;
- problems swallowing;
- coughing or choking;
- gurgling or a wet voice after swallowing;
- nasal regurgitation;
- feeling that the food 'becomes stuck' or is 'held up';

- pushing the plate away. However, dysphagia is not the only cause of appetite loss in stroke survivors.

Persistent dysphagia can cause aspiration – breathing food, saliva, liquids or vomit into the lungs. This encourages the growth of bacteria, leading to pneumonia (infection of the lungs). So, if you suspect that you or the person you care for has dysphagia, ask your GP for a referral to a speech and language therapist or a dietician experienced in assessing swallowing problems.

Helping food go down

A dietician can work out a meal plan that is easy to swallow. For example:

- Minced, mashed and pureed food can compensate for fatigue, chewing and swallowing problems. You can buy 'ready meals' prepared for people with swallowing problems.
- Safely swallowing water, tea and other thin liquids requires particularly fine coordination. Adding thick-

Table 3 Safe swallowing tips

Do not mix food and drink in the same mouthful
Do not talk while you are eating
Keep each mouthful small: this may mean you only eat or drink a teaspoon's worth at a time
Sit upright for half an hour after each meal
Swallow each mouthful before eating or drinking any more
Take your time; mealtimes should be relaxed and quiet
Try eating smaller meals more frequently, rather than three larger meals a day

Source: Adapted from the Stroke Association

eners to water, juice and other thin drinks, carbonation or changing the temperature may help.

Follow the safe swallowing tips (Table 3) and ask your occupational therapist for the best position in which to eat. Speech and language therapists can teach alternative swallowing manoeuvres and suggest exercises to improve swallowing tailored to your problems.

Movement problems

Almost nine in every ten people who experience an ischaemic stroke develop motor (movement) problems including:

- hemiplegia – weaknesses on one side of the body;
- hemiballism – vigorous, irregular and marked limb movements on one side of the body that typically develop around the time of the stroke;
- chorea – brief, non-repetitive movements that appear to move from muscle to muscle;
- spasticity – abnormal increase in muscle tone;
- dystonia – involuntary sustained twisting, repetitive movements or abnormal postures. Dystonia tends to emerge, on average, 9.5 months after the stroke but it can emerge up to three years later. People with hemiplegia often develop dystonia once their muscle strength begins to recover.

Survivors should, in general, begin to get back on their feet within 24 hours of the stroke. Immobility, even for a short time, can increase the risk of, for example, muscle wastage, movement problems, slow wound healing, problems urinating and pressure sores.

Treating movement disorders

As many people need help getting around, at least in the short term, the rehabilitation team will train carers in, for example, safely moving the survivor – such as getting out of bed or getting up from a chair. The team will also make sure the carer and survivor can use assistance devices.

The therapist may also:

- stimulate affected muscles with a mild electrical current;
- use certain drugs;
- provide a mitt that you wear over your good hand, thus forcing you to use the 'weak' hand;
- use splints and other externally applied devices (orthoses) to improve function and movement, or reduce pain;
- suggest computer-controlled automated devices that can move a limb – essentially robots – which

Splints

A splint or orthosis can increase your range of movement if, for example, your muscles and tendons permanently shorten (contracture). Ankle–foot orthoses or strapping help maintain your stability. Hand and wrist splints can help you grip, allow you or your carer to reach your palm to make sure it is clean, and stop your fingernails from digging into your palm.

You or your family should know how and when to remove the splint or orthosis and watch for redness and other signs of skin damage. Broken skin can develop into an open sore that is often very hard to heal.

can help, for example, while relearning grasping skills or offering additional support. The use of robotic and related technology by stroke survivors is likely to grow.

Falls

About two-fifths of stroke survivors fall at least once during rehabilitation. So, survivors are about seven times more likely to break a bone in the year after the stroke compared to the general population. Certain stroke survivors seem especially likely to fall, including those with hemi-neglect (see 'Vision', page 40) or movement problems. Some anticoagulants and a lack of weight-bearing by a disabled limb weaken the bones, which increases fracture risk. Carers need to know how to prevent falls, how to help someone up and how to adapt the home.

Spasticity

Each muscle has two sets of nerves. One set tells muscles to contact. The other tells the muscle to relax. If a stroke damages signals telling the muscles to con-tract, limbs may be limp, flaccid and floppy. If a stroke damages the signals telling the muscles to relax, limbs may become stiff and show involuntary muscle spasms (spasticity). Muscles that stay contracted can pull joints into abnormal positions or prevent normal motion.

Stroke survivors may also show rapid muscle contractions (clonus), exaggerated reflexes, muscle spasms, scissoring (involuntary crossing of the legs) and 'locked' joints. Untreated, muscles affected by spasticity can develop contracture. Treating spasticity usually includes physical therapy and, in some cases, ice massage, heat packs, surgery and drugs that relax muscle. Botulinum toxin – Botox – injections relax muscle and improve tone.

Vision

Stroke survivors may experience problems with sight – including double vision, blurred vision, poor depth perception and nystagmus (continuous, uncontrolled eye movement). Hemianopia – loss of the visual field (how much you can see at any time) on one side of the body – can lead to difficulty balancing or with coordination, as well as problems recognizing things or people and reading.

Strokes may also lead to difference in awareness between the two sides of the body (hemi-neglect). Doctors can test for hemi-neglect by asking the survivor to cross out lines on a page, draw a clock, copy a figure or mark the centre of a line. Hemi-neglect does not necessarily arise from damage to the brain's visual areas. Damage to areas that receive and process signals from the eye may mean the person 'sees' the side but does not 'know' that he or she sees it.

Physiotherapists and occupational therapists can help you compensate. For example:

- 'Vision exploration training' can help survivors develop strategies to search a visual field. Just moving the head from side to side helps scan areas on the 'damaged' side.
- A clinical psychologist can suggest ways to, for example, recognize things or people.
- An ophthalmologist or optician can offer visual aids, such as spectacles that help compensate for hemi-neglect.

- Try large print books and audio books.
- Brightly coloured lines or running a highlighter along the edge of the page can draw attention to the neglected side.
- If people cannot perceive items on one side, place the most important items for a task – such as clothes – on the other side.

Incontinence and urinary problems

About four-fifths of survivors experience urinary incontinence at least for a short time after their stroke. Some do not get to the toilet in time. Some make it in time but feel a desperate need to pass urine (so-called urgency) or a need to pass urine often (frequency). Many stroke survivors also have faecal incontinence.

Bladder and bowel control usually improves over time, but about one in five survivors have urinary incontinence six months after their stroke. Some

---

Some causes of incontinence after a stroke

These may include:

- damage to the nerves or brain areas controlling the bladder and bowel;
- changes in diet;
- being bedbound;
- difficulty communicating to carers that the person needs to use the toilet;
- mobility problems;
- brain damage that means the person is less aware that he or she needs to go to the toilet;
- certain medicines.

people who cannot pass water properly need a catheter inserted into their bladder. Because a catheter increases the risk of infections and other complications, doctors will leave this in for the shortest time possible.

There's lots of help available – so ask:

- A specialist nurse, called a continence adviser, can suggest aids, such as pads and bed covers, and teach exercises that strengthen muscles around the bladder and urethra. These exercises help you hold on until you reach the toilet.
- Physiotherapists can improve your mobility and so help you use the toilet or commode.
- Occupational therapists may be able to suggest adaptations that make using the toilet easier, such as making the seat higher.
- Doctors can prescribe drugs that help with some types of urinary incontinence.
- Reducing the amount of caffeine you drink may help. Drink plain water, fruit juices and herbal teas instead.

Watch for urinary tract infections

A quarter of stroke survivors develop a urinary tract infection (UTI). You are three to four times more likely to develop a UTI if you have a catheter. See your GP if you develop any of the following:

- urinary incontinence or you cannot urinate;
- you urinate much more or less often than usual;
- urination hurts or your lower back hurts;
- change in the colour of your urine – such as being bloody or brown;
- urine that smells;

- urine that seems to have a different consistency from usual;
- urine that contains a sediment;
- other signs of an infection, such as chills or a fever.

Pain

Pain is common after a stroke. For example:

- Strokes affecting parts of the brain that process pain cause 'central pain', which typically emerges several weeks or months later. Commonly, the damage exaggerates stimulation in a weakened part of a body: a light touch evokes a searing, burning, itching or stretching pain. While conventional painkillers are often ineffective, pregabalin and gabapentin (also used to treat epilepsy) often help.
- Problems with muscles and joints (for example, spasticity or changes in gait) and depression can trigger or exacerbate pain.
- Many survivors experience headaches, especially following haemorrhagic strokes. The cause is unclear, although painkillers often help.

Try to communicate the severity and site of your pain. But communication and cognitive difficulties can make this difficult. So, carers and healthcare professionals should ask specifically about pain.

Seizures and epilepsy

Up to one in ten stroke survivors experience seizure disorders after a stroke. Indeed, strokes are the most common reason why seizures emerge for the first time in elderly people. In a few cases, you may need to take anticonvulsants.

Seizures arise from bouts of uncontrolled electrical activity in the brain. This causes tingling and twitching in, for example, an arm or a leg. The classic seizures – a 'grand mal' or tonic–clonic seizure, in which someone loses consciousness and twitches uncontrollably on the ground – are rare after a stroke unless the person previously had epilepsy.

A seizure is one of the first symptoms of about 1 in 50 strokes. However, a brain tumour, withdrawal from alcohol and drugs, an abscess in the brain and other conditions can also cause seizures, which can complicate diagnosis. In addition, some seizure disorders can mimic strokes.

6

Lifestyle changes to prevent another stroke

The Kitava people of Papua New Guinea follow a traditional subsistence diet and lifestyle. In the early 1990s, researchers could not find a single Kitavan who had suffered a stroke. Indeed, none of the Kitavans could recall anyone dying with symptoms suggesting a stroke. Closer to home, the traditional Mediterranean diet protects against stroke. This:

- is rich in olive oil and canola (rapeseed) oil;
- is low in cholesterol and saturated (animal) fat;
- contains large amounts of whole grains, fruit, vegetables, lentils, beans and nuts; and
- uses fish rather than red meat.

Cooking safely after a stoke

Cooking can be difficult and dangerous after a stroke. Memory problems may mean that survivors wander off while cooking. Weakness or poor dexterity can make moving pots, plates and pans difficult and survivors may spill hot food or drink. Your occupational therapist can suggest changes that make cooking easier and safer, including sliding rather than lifting pans, splatter screens and, if you use a wheelchair, a mirror that can help you see into the pans. A hotplate, microwave and toaster oven may be safer than a conventional cooker.

During the first few weeks and months after a stroke, your dietician will suggest a diet to aid your recovery. Once you have recovered, healthy eating, quitting smoking and controlling alcohol consumption can help prevent another stroke. And healthy eating helps prevent the first stroke or TIA.

Reducing salt

Each 5 grams of salt you eat each day increases stroke risk by about a quarter. So, follow your doctor's or dietician's advice: some people need to eat less than the general recommendation (6 grams a day).

Crisps and peanuts taste salty. However, many foods contain surprisingly large amounts of hidden salt including some, bread, biscuits, processed meat, cheese, stock cubes and even ice cream. So read the label and:

- avoid foods – such as smoked meat and fish – that are high in salt;
- add as little salt as you can during baking and cooking;
- banish the salt cellar from the table;
- ask restaurants and take-aways for 'no salt';
- use low-salt ketchup, pickles, mustard, yeast extract, stock cubes and so on;
- avoid foods that include a chemical name that includes sodium, such as disodium phosphate, monosodium glutamate or sodium nitrate;
- Choose meals and sandwiches with less than 1.25 grams of salt per meal.
- Choose individual foods – such as soups and sauces – with less than 0.75 grams of salt per serving.

Stroke sometimes causes profound problems with smell and taste. So, some survivors begin adding unhealthy amounts of salt to their food to improve the taste. One woman added up to 110 grams of salt a day to her food to stop it tasting bland. Instead of reaching for the salt cellar, learn how to use herbs and spices.

Fruit and vegetables

A diet rich in fruit and vegetables can cut stroke risk by around a fifth (Table 4). So, eat at least five portions of

Table 4 Effect of fruit and vegetables on stroke risk

Diet	Reduction in stroke risk
200 grams *more* fruits a day	32 per cent
200 grams *more* vegetables a day	11 per cent
50 grams of fruits a day	10 per cent
400 grams of fruits a day	55 per cent
50 grams of vegetables a day	3 per cent
400 grams of vegetables a day	20 per cent

Table 5 Examples of a portion of fruit and vegetables

One medium-sized fruit (banana, apple, pear, orange)

One slice of a large fruit (melon, pineapple, mango)

Two smaller fruits (plums, satsumas, apricots, peaches)

A dessert bowl full of salad

Three heaped tablespoons of vegetables

Three heaped tablespoons of pulses (chickpeas, lentils, beans)

Two to three tablespoons ('a handful') of grapes or berries

One tablespoon of dried fruit

One glass (150 millilitres) of unsweetened fruit or vegetable juice or smoothie (two or more glasses of juice a day still counts as one portion)

fruit and vegetables a day. (A portion weighs about 80 grams; Table 5.)

A diet rich in fruit and vegetables is high in fibre (roughage), the part of plants that humans cannot digest, such as the outer layers of sweetcorn, beans, wheat and corn. There are two main types:

- Insoluble fibre remains largely intact as it moves through your digestive system and eases defecation. Three-fifths of stroke survivors develop constipation at some time. Some painkillers (especially opioids) can also cause constipation.
- Soluble fibre dissolves in water in the gut, forming a gel that soaks up fats and, in turn, lowers your blood cholesterol levels. Soluble fibre also releases sugar slowly, which staves off hunger pangs and helps you lose weight.

So, eat more oats and oat bran, fruit and vegetables, nuts and seeds, legumes and pulses (such as peas, soya, lentils and chickpeas):

- Whole grains (e.g. wholewheat pasta and whole oats) are an especially rich source of fibre and contain up to 75 per cent more nutrients than refined cereals.
- Peas, lentils, chickpeas and string beans contain up to twice the levels of vitamins and minerals as cereals and are rich in iron, zinc, selenium, magnesium, manganese, copper and nickel.
- Legumes and their seeds (pulses) are high in protein and fibre, and help control levels of fats in the blood.

Protein

Dietary protein reduces stroke risk, in part by lowering blood pressure. People who consume the most protein are typically a fifth less likely to suffer a stroke than those who ate the least, after allowing for other risk factors. The benefit seems to be especially marked against intracerebral haemorrhage: a two-fifths reduction. But avoid fatty cuts of meat.

High levels of LDL (page 16) in the blood increase stroke risk, especially in people who smoke or are inactive. Diet accounts for around a third of the cholesterol in our bodies. The rest comes from saturated fat, which the liver converts into cholesterol. So, choose the leanest cuts of meat, trim any visible fat and do not eat chicken skin, pork crackling or bacon rind. If changing to a low-fat diet does not reduce your blood cholesterol level sufficiently, you may need to take medicines. However, these are an addition to a low-fat diet, not a replacement.

Fish and omega-3 fatty acids

Fish are rich in omega-3 fatty acids, also called omega-3 polyunsaturated fatty acids (PUFAs). Among other actions, omega-3 PUFAs reduce blood pressure, improve levels of cholesterol and other fats in your blood and optimize platelet (page 26) function – all of which reduce stroke risk. Omega-3 PUFAs are also important for memory, intellectual performance and healthy vision, which a stroke may affect. Eating oily fish also keeps joints healthy. Rehabilitation can place extra stresses and strains on your joints.

Humans can make omega-3 fatty acids from another fat in green leafy vegetables, nuts, seeds and their oils.

But it is a slow process. So, the UK's stroke guidance suggests eating two portions of oily fish each week (e.g. salmon, trout, herring, pilchards, sardines or fresh tuna). If you eat canned fish, check the label to make sure processing has not depleted the omega-3 oils. If at first you do not like the taste of oily fish, do not give up without trying some different sources and a few recipes. There are plenty of suggestions on the internet (for example, see <www.thefishsociety.co.uk>) and in cookbooks.

Exercise

The Stroke Association notes that even moderate exercise reduces stroke risk by more than a quarter. Yet two in every five survivors do not get out as much as they would like.

The UK's stroke guidance suggests taking at least 2.5 hours of moderate-intensity exercise each week in bouts of at least ten minutes. At least twice per week, stroke survivors should take part in activities that strengthen muscles and, if you are at risk of falls, improve balance and coordination.

Start gently – for example, a very short walk or a few minutes on an exercise bike or a slow treadmill. Then slowly increase the time. However, check the exercise regimen with your GP or stroke team before starting. Stop exercising and seek medical help immediately if you experience any of the following:

- chest pain or angina;
- light-headedness;
- confusion;
- cold or clammy skin.

Try to make exercise part of your everyday life, such as:

- walking to the local shops;
- riding a bike to work;
- parking a 15-minute walk from your place of work;
- getting off the bus, tube or train one or two stops early;
- using the stairs instead of the lift;
- cleaning the house regularly;
- washing your car by hand;
- growing your own vegetables and gardening;
- taking your dog for more walks.

Ask your occupational therapist or physiotherapist about footwear. Most stroke survivors prefer training shoes or flat supportive shoes with ankle support when walking. Loose clothes – such as jogging clothes – help ensure you have sufficient movement.

Try to get out of town. Japanese people with long-term illnesses often walk in woods – called *shinrin-yoku* (forest bathing) – which, among other benefits, encourages relaxation, reduces stress, lowers blood pressure and boosts the immune system. So, make the most of our country parks and nature reserves. If you are worried about tripping and falling, stick to those with prepared paths.

Drink to your health?

People who regularly consume large amounts of alcohol are three times more likely to suffer a stroke compared to teetotallers, the Stroke Association warns. If you have suffered a stroke or TIA or have another health problem, you should follow your doctor's advice.

Tips to cut down

Most people want to tackle their drinking themselves before seeing a doctor or joining a support group such as Alcoholics Anonymous (<www.alcoholics-anonymous.org.uk>). So, note how much you drink and when (places and circumstances – such as when you are feeling down or stressed out) over a month. Don't guess. Alcohol Concern (<www.alcoholconcern.org.uk>) says the average adult drinker underestimates consumption by the equivalent of a bottle of wine a week. If you get so drunk that you cannot recall how much you drank, you have a problem. In addition, people who abuse alcohol tend to drink more regularly than other drinkers, in some cases to stave off withdrawal symptoms, such as shakes, insomnia, agitation and depression.

Set a goal. (If you have survived a stroke, speak to your doctor first.) Some people will need to abstain. Others can drink within the recommended limit – but they need to remain alert for changes in their drinking habits. Even if you plan to return to drinking safe levels of alcohol, it is worth 'drying out' for at least a month to allow your body to recover. If you cannot stop drinking for a few weeks, you probably have an alcohol problem. Take milk thistle to help your liver recover (check with your doctor or pharmacist first if you are taking other medicines).

Various tricks can help you reduce your consumption of alcohol:

- Replace large glasses with smaller ones.
- Use a spirit measure at home.
- Drink alcohol only with a meal.
- Look at the label and avoid wine with an alcohol by volume (ABV) of 14 or 15 per cent.

- Alternate alcoholic beverages with water or soft drinks.
- Mix your drink – try spritzers and shandies rather than plain wine and beer.
- Quench your thirst with a soft drink.
- Make sure you have 'dry' days each week. You may need to avoid your usual haunts and drinking partners.
- Find a hobby that does not involve drinking.
- Avoid buying rounds, which can rapidly rack up the amount you consume.
- Ask for bottles of beer, shandies and spritzers, or halves instead of pints.

Deciding whether to tell your family, friends and colleagues that you are cutting down can be difficult. Some family and friends offer advice and support. Others may feel that you are challenging their drinking habits – and may prove hostile or condescending, especially if some of your social life or occupation revolves around drinking. You could offer to be the designated driver or tell a white lie and claim that your doctor has advised you not to drink.

If you feel you really cannot quit without help, your doctor can refer you to NHS alcohol services or offer drugs to help you deal with cravings. Cognitive behavioural therapists and counsellors can help you understand why you drink, offer suggestions to help you cut down and deal with difficult situations. Many people find hypnotism helps. If you drink to cope with pain, depression or anxiety your doctor can suggest painkillers, counselling and medicines.

The healthy alternative

Dehydration is common after a stroke, partly because of swallowing problems, partly because survivors often rely on other people to get them a drink and partly because the stroke may reduce sensitivity to thirst. Even in healthy people, mild dehydration can cause, for example:

- constipation;
- increased risk of DVT;
- reduced vigilance and concentration;
- poor memory;
- increased tension or anxiety;
- fatigue;
- headache.

The NHS notes that adults should drink 1.2 litres of water (six to eight glasses) each day to replace fluids lost in urine, sweat and so on. If you feel thirsty for long periods, you are not drinking enough. Increase your intake during exercise or hot weather (or in a hot ward), if you feel lightheaded, pass dark-coloured urine or have not passed urine within six hours. See your doctor if you regularly feel thirsty despite maintaining your fluid intake. Excessive thirst can be a symptom of diabetes.

Quit smoking

Smokers are about three times to suffer a stroke than non-smokers. People who smoke 20 cigarettes a day are six times more likely to have a stroke. Unfortunately, on some measures, nicotine is more addictive than heroin or cocaine. As a result, fewer than one smoker in 30 quits each year and more than half of those who quit relapse within a year, partly because of the withdrawal symptoms, which can leave you irritable, restless, anxious, sleepless and intensely craving a cigarette.

Withdrawal generally abates over about two weeks. If you cannot tough it out, nicotine replacement therapy (NRT) 'tops up' levels in the blood, without exposing you to the other harmful chemicals. So, NRT can alleviate the withdrawal symptoms and increase your chances of quitting by between 50 and 100 per cent. You can choose from various types of NRT:

- Patches reduce withdrawal symptoms over a relatively long time, but start alleviating symptoms relatively slowly.
- Nicotine chewing gum, lozenges, inhalers and nasal sprays act more quickly but the effect is shorter lived than a patch.

The power of hypnosis

Doctors still do not understand fully how hypnotism works. However, essentially, hypnosis is focused attention and concentration. Some hypnotists describe the process as like losing track of what's going on when you are lost in a book or movie. Hypnosis may help control pain, alleviate stress and change harmful habits such as abusing alcohol, comfort eating or smoking. Hypnosis can increase the chances of quitting smoking almost fivefold, for example. A hypnotist cannot make you do or say anything he or she wants and you will be able to come 'out' of hypnosis whenever you want. Numerous self-hypnosis DVDs, CDs and books help you create the 'focused attention' that underpins hypnosis. Contact the British Association of Medical Hypnosis (<www.bamh.org.uk/>).

Talk to your pharmacist or GP to find the right combination. Doctors can prescribe other treatments. While these offer a helping hand, you still need to be motivated to quit.

Many people have quit using e-cigarettes. These don't contain the cancer-causing chemicals laden in tobacco smoke. But as e-cigarettes deliver nicotine, they remain addictive and we still don't know if there are any long-term health risks. Nevertheless, e-cigarettes are far safer than conventional tobacco and can take you a large step towards kicking the habit, but don't stop there.

Lose weight

Being overweight increases the risk of an ischaemic stroke by a fifth, according to the Stroke Association. Being obese increases the risk by more than half. Indeed, overweight people are likely to have several stroke risk factors, including high cholesterol, hypertension and diabetes.

Nevertheless, weight is not a very good guide to your risk of developing stroke and other diseases. Weighing 14 stone (89 kg) is fine if you are 6 foot 5 inches (1.96 m). But you'd be seriously obese if you weigh 14 stone and you're 5 foot 6 inches (1.68 m). BMI takes your height and weight into account and so offers a better indication of whether you are overweight; see <www.nhs. uk/ Tools/Pages/Healthyweightcalculator.aspx>.

- The ideal BMI is between 18.5 and 24.9 kg/m^2. Below this and you are dangerously underweight.
- A BMI between 25.0 and 29.9 kg/m^2 suggests that you are overweight.
- You are probably obese if your BMI exceeds 30.0 kg/m^2.

Table 6 Waist sizes linked to health risk

	Health at risk by waist size	Health at high risk by waist size
Men	Over 94 centimetres (37 inches)	Over 102 centimetres (40 inches)
Women	Over 80 centimetres (32 inches)	Over 88 centimetres (35 inches)
South Asian men		Over 90 centimetres (36 inches)
South Asian women		Over 80 centimetres (32 inches)

Source: Adapted from the British Heart Foundation

BMI may overestimate body fat in athletes, body-builders and other muscular people and underestimate body fat in older persons and people who have lost muscle, which can happen after a stroke. Doctors and gyms can measure your body fat. However, abdominal obesity damages your health more than fat elsewhere, especially in people of South Asian descent, who are more likely to have a stroke than Caucasians (Table 6).

Tips to help you lose weight

- Record everything you eat and drink for a couple of weeks. The odd biscuit, the extra glass of wine or full-fat latte soon adds up. You can also see if you are eating fatty or high-salt food.
- Set a realistic, specific target based on your BMI, such as to lose 2 stone (about 12.5 kilograms) by Christmas. Cutting 500 to 1,000 calories each day

can reduce weight by between 0.5 and 1.0 kilograms each week.

- Think about how you tried to lose weight in the past. What techniques and diets worked? Which failed to make a difference? Did a support group help?
- Do not let a slip-up derail your diet. Try to identify why you indulged.
- Begin your diet when you are at home over a weekend or a holiday and you do not have a celebration (such as Christmas or a birthday) planned. It is tougher changing your diet on a Monday morning or in a hotel faced with fat-laden food, caffeine-rich drinks and alcohol.
- Talk to your GP or pharmacist. Several medicines may help kick-start your weight loss. But make sure they know that you have had a stroke and any medicines you're taking.

If you are recovering from a stroke, ask your dietician or stroke team what your ideal weight should be and when to start dieting.

7

Life after a stroke

Strokes strike suddenly, giving you and your family very little time to prepare for life with the problems that can follow. Your rehabilitation team will offer you tailored advice. But don't overestimate your or, if you are a carer, the survivor's abilities. If you as a carer feel – or the stroke survivor insists – that he or she can do a task, remain with the person until you are sure he or she is safe. If you are a survivor, remember that allowing your carer to help helps your carer. Carers report better psychological well-being when they provide more assistance.

Reducing the risk of falls

Stroke survivors may be especially vulnerable to falls and broken bones. For example, a person with cognitive problems may take unnecessary risks. You can make your home safer. Many of these suggestions are sensible for older people generally:

- An occupational therapist, physiotherapist or social worker can suggest mobility aids (such as walking sticks or a wheelchair). However, even 'simple' walking sticks need to be appropriate for your height and weight.
- Ramps, handrails and grab bars at home reduce the risk of falls.

- Avoid badly fitting or inappropriate footwear.
- Don't rush.
- If you are buying carpet, get one with a short pile. People with a cane, walker or wheelchair can find longer piles difficult to move around on.
- Tuck extension cables and leads away.
- Ensure there is good lighting inside and outside the house.
- Stick down loose carpets and mats, and limit clutter.

Using a bathroom

An accessible bathroom can help people keep clean without asking for help, which bolsters their self-esteem. Several simple adaptations can make a big difference:

- Liquid soap or a washcloth pouch can be easier to handle than a bar of soap.
- Putting sponge, plastic or foam around the base of hairbrushes, toothbrushes and bottles helps grip.
- Toothpaste pumps are often easier to use than a tube.
- Try electric razors rather than blades.
- Try long-handled sponges.
- A seat or bench in the shower or bath can help people who are experiencing problems with balance, perception or strength.
- A rubber mat or decals can prevent slipping in the bath.

Making dressing easier

- Wear loose clothing that closes at the front.
- Wear trousers and skirts with elastic waistbands.
- Lay clothes out in the order you put them on.
- Get dressed and undressed while sitting on the bed or on a chair.
- Put clothes on to your weak or disabled arm or leg first. Undress in the same order.
- If needed, use a buttonhook or Velcro. Button clothes from the bottom up.
- Bright prints and complex patterns can confuse people with visual or perceptual problems. Buy solid colours and simple designs instead.
- Attach a metal key ring loop to zips. Do any buttons up before using the zip.
- Occupational therapists may be able to teach people to dress one-handed.

Living with fatigue

Post-stroke fatigue is not like 'normal' tiredness. You may lack the energy to shop, use the telephone, care for yourself or participate in your exercises, therapy or rehabilitation. You may need to rest every day or almost every day. However, rest may not improve the fatigue. 'Soldiering on' just makes matters worse.

In the weeks and months after a stroke, fatigue can arise because your body is healing, rehabilitation can burn off a lot of energy, and you have probably lost stamina and fitness. Over the longer term, a disability can make walking and other 'normal' activities more tiring. Several other factors can exacerbate fatigue, including:

Tips for a good night's sleep for you and your carer

- Try not to brood on problems, which makes them seem worse, exacerbates stress, keeps you awake and, because you are tired in the morning, means you are less able to deal with your difficulties. Avoid heavy discussions before bed.
- Do not worry about anything you have forgotten to do. Jot it down (you could keep a notepad by the bed) and try to forget about the problem until the morning.
- Go to bed at the same time each night and set your alarm for the same time each morning, even at the weekends. This helps re-establish a regular sleep pattern.
- Avoid naps during the day.
- Avoid stimulants, such as caffeine and nicotine, for several hours before bed. Try hot milk or milky drinks instead.
- Do not drink too much fluid (even non-alcoholic) just before bed as this can mean regular trips to the bathroom.
- Avoid alcohol. A nightcap can help you fall asleep, but as blood levels of alcohol fall, sleep becomes more fragmented and lighter. So, you may wake repeatedly.
- Do not eat a heavy meal before bedtime.
- Although regular exercise helps you sleep, exercising just before bed can disrupt sleep.
- Use the bed for sex and sleep only. Do not work or watch TV in bed.
- Invest in a comfortable mattress, with enough bedclothes. Make sure the room is not too hot, too cold or too bright.
- If you cannot sleep, get up and watch TV or read – nothing too stimulating – until you feel tired. Lying there worrying about not sleeping just keeps you awake.

- the stroke itself, although doctors do not understand why;
- depression and anxiety;
- some medicines: check with your doctor as there are often alternatives;
- insomnia and sleep disturbances caused by pain;
- breathing problems;
- eating problems and poor nutrition.

Give yourself plenty of time, don't try to do too much too soon, pace yourself and take breaks. The improvement in fatigue is likely to be gradual and your energy will probably wax and wane. You could keep a diary of your activities each day, which will remind you of your progress and help you find the right balance of activity and rest. If you are having a good day, stick to your plans. If you do too much too soon, you may feel exhausted for the next couple of days. Nevertheless, gradually increasing the amount that you exercise may help reduce tiredness.

Dealing with emotional and psychiatric problems

Coping with the life-changing consequences of a stroke is often devastating for survivors, their partners and their families. Stroke survivors often worry about work, finances and relationships. Many lose confidence. Yet emotional problems are more common than the disability alone can explain. The brain damage that follows a stroke can cause emotional and psychiatric problems.

Depression, for example, is common after a stroke, especially after discharge from hospital. Being back at home highlights the extent of the survivor's disability. Cognitive and communication problems can mean

doctors misdiagnose cognitive problems as depression
and vice versa. Usually, crying and profound sadness
are the most reliable indicators of depression among
stroke survivors. However, therapists can pick up
depression when the person shows poor concentration
or does not progress as expected during rehabilitation.

A survivor with depression is three times more
likely to die in the ten years after the stroke than a
survivor without depression. But the relationship runs
both ways: depression increases stroke risk by about a
third. Several factors probably contribute: depressed
people are more likely to smoke, drink heavily, eat an
unhealthy diet and be physically inactive, for example.
If you feel you have (or someone you care for has)
depression speak to your doctor.

More than depression

In addition to depression, stroke survivors potentially
experience a range of psychological issues, including
anger, helplessness, loss of emotional self-control,
indifference and even euphoria. These changes seem,
in part, to emerge after damage to the parts of the brain
that regulate emotions.

One in five stroke survivors may experience
anxiety, which may emerge several months after the
stroke. Stroke survivors may experience panic attacks
during which they hyperventilate – one manifesta-
tion of anxiety. They may mistake hyperventilation
for another stroke. Some survivors develop phobias
(another type of anxiety) about objects and situations
that they associate with the stroke or around social
situations. Finally, some stroke survivors develop
symptoms of post-traumatic stress disorder (PTSD),
such as flashbacks that emerge 'out of the blue' and

vivid dreams and nightmares. Typically, they avoid places and people that evoke memories of the trauma (such as where they had the stroke), refuse to speak about their experiences and feel constantly on guard or emotionally numb.

If the psychological symptoms markedly affect your daily life, the doctor may suggest antidepressants or drugs to alleviate anxiety (anxiolytics). Drugs do not resolve the underlying problem but may offer a 'window of opportunity' to deal with any issues you face.

Loss of control

Occasionally, survivors develop mania when the stroke damages part of the brain involved in self-control. People with mania seem hyperactive, speak rapidly, have grandiose and unrealistic ideas, cannot sleep, are easily distracted and lack judgement, such as embarking on seemingly ridiculous investments or business schemes.

This loss of self-control can emerge in other ways. For instance, three in every five stroke survivors may exhibit some degree of disinhibition: in other words, they do not follow social rules and conventions. A dis-inhibited person may seem tactless, rude and offensive. About one stroke survivor in ten can become aggressive. Ask the stroke team for advice about responding to inappropriate, distressing or aggressive behaviour.

About a fifth of survivors show emotionalism during the six months after a stroke. These episodes may last up to several minutes and can be distressing and interfere with rehabilitation. About one in ten stroke survivors have long-term emotionalism. Often people with emotionalism stop when you change the subject or call their name. This is not usually the case with depression. Once a doctor has diagnosed emotionalism, you could simply ignore the outburst.

Counselling and cognitive behavioural therapy

Sharing problems, asking for advice or considering a different perspective often helps. Your stroke team, the Stroke Association, your GP or your occupational therapist can put you in touch with, for example, local stroke clubs, counselling, relaxation programmes and exercise groups.

For instance, cognitive behavioural therapy (CBT) identifies the feelings, thoughts and behaviours associated with your stroke or unhealthy lifestyle. The therapist will help you question those feelings, thoughts, behaviours and beliefs. You learn to replace unhelpful and unrealistic behaviours with approaches that actively address problems.

CBT can also use gradual exposure to feared situations or activities, including fears around places and circumstances that you associate with a stroke. During CBT, survivors spend increasing time in situations that they find stressful.

Tensions may also arise because of worries about money or changes in the dynamics of a family's relationships. Again, counselling and other forms of family support might help. It is worth making sure that any counsellor (see <www.bacp.co.uk/>) is familiar with the problems and issues facing stroke survivors and their families.

Getting back to work

Employment (even unpaid) can help recovery from a stroke, protects against depression and anxiety, boosts self-esteem and counters isolation. Of course, paid work also helps financially. Not surprisingly, having relatively intact cognitive abilities and being able to walk increase the chances of returning to work. Yet many people who could work (even part-time and in voluntary roles) do not. (I do not support 'forcing' people who are sick or disabled back to work by attacking benefits. However, helping people back into employment can aid rehabilitation and help get life back to normal.) So, ask your doctor's advice about whether and when you can return to work.

You will need to talk to your employer and colleagues and explain any issues, such as disabilities or fatigue, before you go back. An occupational therapist may need to assess the workplace and help develop a plan that minimizes, for example, physical strain, fatigue and the effect of poor concentration and ascertain whether adapting any equipment or work practices could help. Your GP can refer you to an occupational therapist.

You may need to ease yourself back gently – such as beginning with alternate half-days and working on light or less challenging duties – and gradually build up over several weeks. You may also be able to use advances in IT, such as voice-activated software if you have problems typing, or changing the size of the type on the screen. You might find time management approaches – such as using lists to define your priorities – useful.

Make sure you are aware of the support available. Ask to speak to a medical social worker. If you cannot return to your previous job, you could try, for example, to find charities and non-governmental organizations that would benefit from your experience and that resonate with your interests and beliefs.

Driving after a stroke

Driving helps a stroke survivor get around, boosts self-esteem, self-confidence and mood, and is a tangible sign that life is getting back to normal. But consult your doctor and the Driver and Vehicle Licensing Agency (DVLA) or the Driver and Vehicle Agency (DVA) in Northern Ireland for advice before getting behind the wheel. If the doctor and DVLA or DVA agree you can drive, inform your insurance company.

Sex and the stroke survivor

Stroke survivors and their partners may worry that sex could trigger another stroke. Occasionally, sex triggers an aneurysm to burst. So, people who have survived a haemorrhagic stroke should swallow any embarrassment and check with their doctor before having sex for the first time after the stroke. However, most stroke

Plan holidays carefully

- Check that the accommodation is suitable for your level of disability – such as allowing wheelchair access or not being at the top of a hill.
- Check that the accommodation is not too far from restaurants, shops and entertainment. (Google Maps with Street View may help.)
- Avoid places that are very hot or very cold. Your

cardiovascular system will have to work harder to keep your temperature at the right level.

- Avoid high altitudes when travelling aboard. There is less oxygen in the air at high altitudes. Until you acclimatize your heart has to work harder.
- Try to avoid stress – after all, a holiday is supposed to be a time to relax. You could return to a place you have visited recently to reduce the risk of unwelcome surprises.
- Leave plenty of time to reach the airport or destination.
- Do not carry heavy bags or rush around. People with health problems and disabilities may be able to get transport around the airport, ferry terminal or port.
- Check with your GP or rehabilitation team (as well as the airline and travel insurance company) that it is safe to fly.
- Check that your travel insurance offers adequate coverage.
- Ensure you have information about local emergency and health services in your destination – ask your tour operator or, in the UK, use NHS Choices.
- Check that you take sufficient medicines – a repeat prescription will not be available at the end of a phone. Have a supply of your medicines in your hand luggage and in your suitcase, and take a list of all your drugs and doses if you need to visit an accident and emergency department or see an unfamiliar doctor.
- Check for any restrictions about bringing medicines (bought from a pharmacy or on prescription) into your destination. Some countries ban certain painkillers that are widely available in the UK, for example. Check with the relevant consulate or embassy.

survivors can restart their sex life without worries. Sometimes the increased opportunities to be close to, and intimate with, a partner increase sexual desire.

However, many stroke survivors do not feel sexually desirable. Depression, stress and certain medications may cause or contribute to erectile dysfunction, vaginal dryness and other sexual problems. (Your doctor can often suggest an alternative.) A male partner of a survivor can also develop erectile dysfunction. For example, he may be afraid he will hurt his partner. Some stroke survivors may not feel desire for a partner who has taken on more of a caring role.

Talking to the stroke team, a counsellor or a patient support group often helps find a way around the problem. The Stroke Association also produces a range of helpful leaflets. But never buy or use any treatment for impotence – whether a herbal remedy or bought on-line – without speaking to your doctor.

Stroke, your family and friends

Caring for a stroke survivor can be tough. Spouses often shoulder considerable responsibility for implementing and supporting lifestyle changes and rehabilitation. There will probably be times when the survivor does not seem to make progress or even appears to go backwards. So, remain positive and offer encouragement. Carers need to walk a tightrope between helping and allowing the survivor to regain his or her independence and self-esteem.

Some carers need to balance a job or childcare with looking after a stroke survivor, which can cause considerable stress. Your relationships and roles can change fundamentally. Children or spouses may find themselves in a parental role. Stroke survivors may feel helpless and dependent. They may live overshadowed by stress and practical problems, be afraid of dying and feel upset at not being able to take part in previously enjoyed activities. Try to understand what the stroke survivor is going through – talk to him or her, speak to patient organizations, and attend support meetings or stroke clubs. The Stroke Association offers family support services in some parts of the country.

Not surprisingly, many survivors feel depressed, angry, guilty and bad-tempered, which can place a strain on your relationships. From time to time, carers feel frustrated, angry, resentful and even depressed. Other family members may feel they do not receive sufficient attention. Do not bottle these feelings up. Talk to your partner, friends and family, carers of other stroke survivors or a counsellor. Carers Direct is a national information, advice and support service for carers in England (<www.nhs.uk/carersdirect>; tel. 0808 802 0202).

Carers report better psychological well-being when they are in better physical health. So look after yourself. Try to unwind while your partner is resting and get a good night's sleep. Do not feel guilty about taking time out for yourself. Carers who participate in the activities that they value feel they have greater control over their life, gain more from providing care and report better physical health and psychological well-being than those who give up activities that they once valued.

Fewer people than a generation ago experience a stroke, and the chances of surviving and making a full recovery are better than ever. Nevertheless, someone in the UK suffers a stroke every five minutes and one in five proves fatal. And despite the medical progress, you cannot rely on drugs and surgery to save your life. But we have seen throughout this book that you and your carer can still live full and rich lives. I wish you both well.